DR. KATHLEEN STAMBAUGH

The Revolution in Teeth Replacement

What Patients Need to Know Before Having Dental Implants

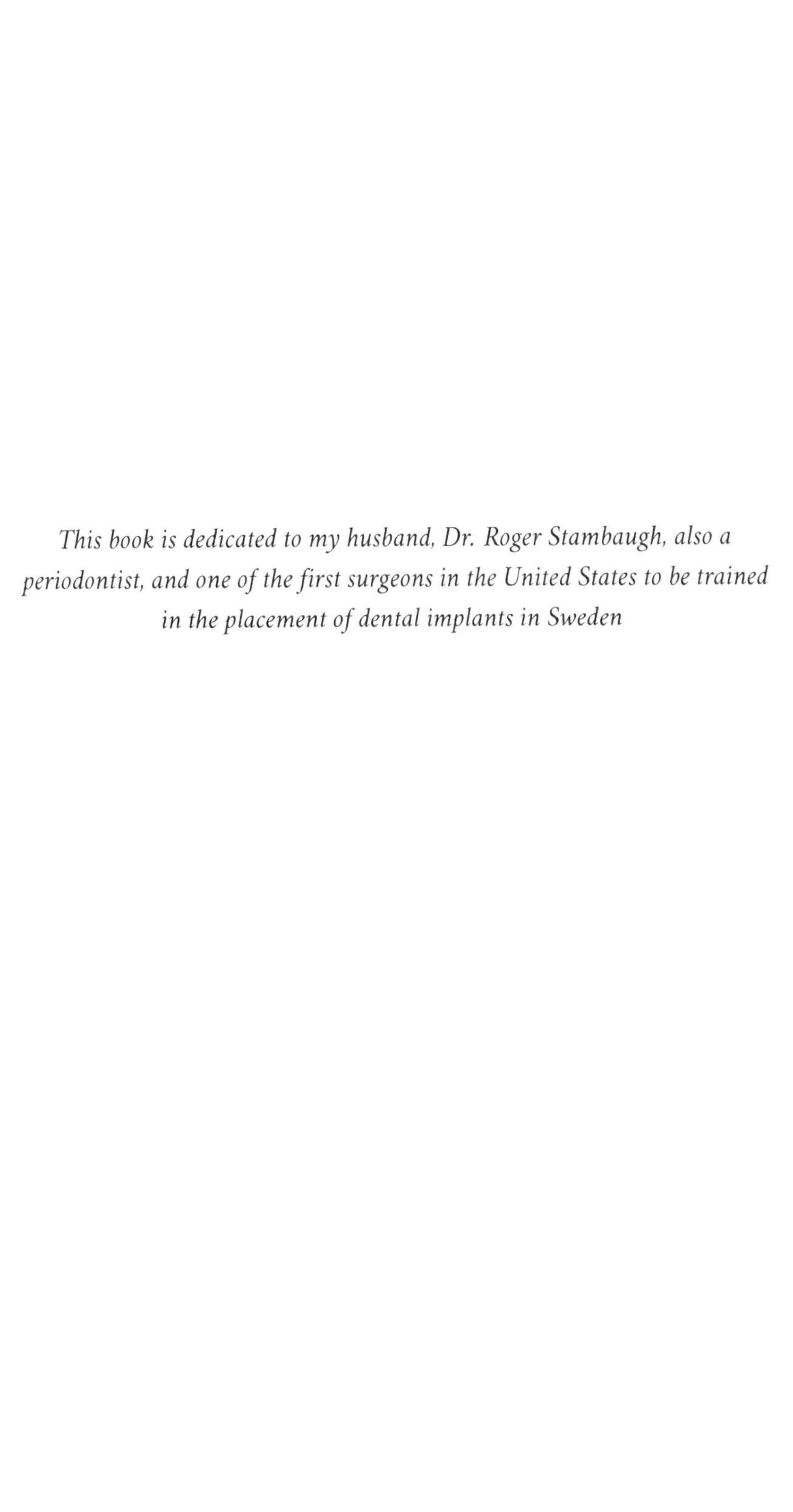

This book is dedicated to my husband, Dr. Roger Stambaugh, also a periodontist, and one of the first surgeons in the United States to be trained in the placement of dental implants in Sweden

Contents

1

Introduction

Most people have heard of dental implants or may even know someone who has them. The purpose of this book is to educate patients who are missing teeth, in terms of what the options are for teeth replacement. I am a periodontist, that is, a dentist specialized in treating gum infections by non-surgical and surgical means, regenerating supporting bone around teeth when possible, performing plastic surgery of the gums, performing esthetic gum surgery to improve appearance of the smile, and replacement of missing teeth with dental implants. For over 35 years, my main focus has been to save patients' natural teeth and establish oral health by eliminating gum infections. When this is not possible, due to advanced bone loss from infection, tooth fracture, or trauma, other options must be considered, one of which is surgical placement of dental implants. I will also be educating the reader about non-implant options for teeth replacement, but the main focus of this publication is to provide a good overview of implant options so that good decisions may be made.

One may think, why is it necessary to replace missing teeth (other than wisdom teeth)? If the missing tooth is the very back molar, it may not be necessary to replace it, if function is still good with the remaining teeth. Some patients can get along with bicuspid function, that is, not having molars. A typical quadrant (quarter of the mouth) starting in the back, will have two molars, two bicuspids, one canine, and two incisors. If the missing tooth however, is between natural teeth, leaving a space, it is best to replace it for a few reasons. First, is that when a space is left between natural teeth, the remaining teeth will likely drift and/or rotate and may ultimately interfere with the proper relationship between upper and lower teeth. Drifting of teeth will open up spaces for food impaction and can be negative in terms of esthetics (appearance). It is important to maintain proper contact between teeth to preserve the stability of the other teeth present.

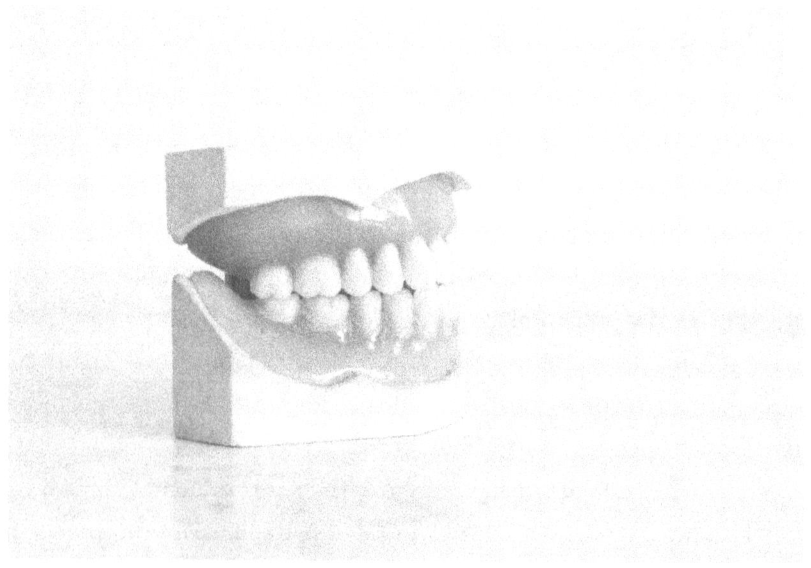

Photo of upper and lower dentures (constructed of pink plastic to

**mimic the gums and plastic or porcelain teeth). This illustrates
the full complement of 28 teeth.**

To begin, I will first briefly define what a dental implant is. Essentially, a dental implant may be thought of as a tooth root replacement. It is surgically placed into the patient's jawbone where the tooth is missing. The "tooth" or "teeth" is/are attached to the implant(s) in a separate procedure usually after initial healing of the implant(s). The tooth part or "crown" is connected to the implant by means of an intervening part called an abutment.

A dental implant is composed of medical grade titanium the majority of the time and is essentially a medical device that mimics a natural tooth root, but with some differences from natural teeth. One implant company (Straumann) also uses a titanium-zirconium alloy which allows faster healing. There are also metal-free ceramic zirconia implants which are whitish in color. This could be an advantage in situations where the gum tissue is extremely thin, so that the grayness of the titanium metal does not show through the thin gum tissue. The shape of all implants is similar to a tube and it is round at the level of the bone. Natural teeth are not perfectly round, and have different shapes and sizes, depending upon their location in the mouth: top or bottom, front or back. Implants do come in various widths and lengths, but they are essentially round at the level of the bone. The implants fuse directly to the bone, a process defined as osseointegration, whereas natural teeth are connected to bone by fibrous periodontal ligaments, which allow slight movement of the teeth with function. This is an important distinction which will become obvious later.

In the following text, I will make reference to implant(s) either singular or plural. The information I present may be implied to both.

2

History

B**rief History of Modern Dental Implants - 55 years ago**

Modern dental implants were first introduced in Sweden by Professor Brànemark, an orthopedic surgeon. The discovery that titanium could help patients who were missing teeth was serendipitous. Dr. Brànemark was performing research on new blood vessel formation in living rabbits' bones. He used optical chambers that were inserted into the rabbits' bones which had been housed in titanium through which he could view blood vessel formation during healing.

When Dr. Brànemark later went to retrieve the titanium-housed chambers for reuse, he had great difficulty getting them out of the bone; they were fused directly to the bone. This became of interest to the dental department, which had numerous patients missing most of their teeth. The first modern dental implants were used to support removable dentures. This greatly improved the function for these patients. The success rate in this Swedish group of patients was very high. Surgeons from the United States (oral surgeons and periodontists) were first trained in the placement of dental implants by the Brånemark group in Sweden.

The United States has become a leader in implant restorations since they were first placed in the U.S. Now, implants are used most commonly to replace teeth in a fixed (non-removable) fashion, so they have progressed from support of removable dentures alone to primarily non-removable replacement of single or multiple teeth.

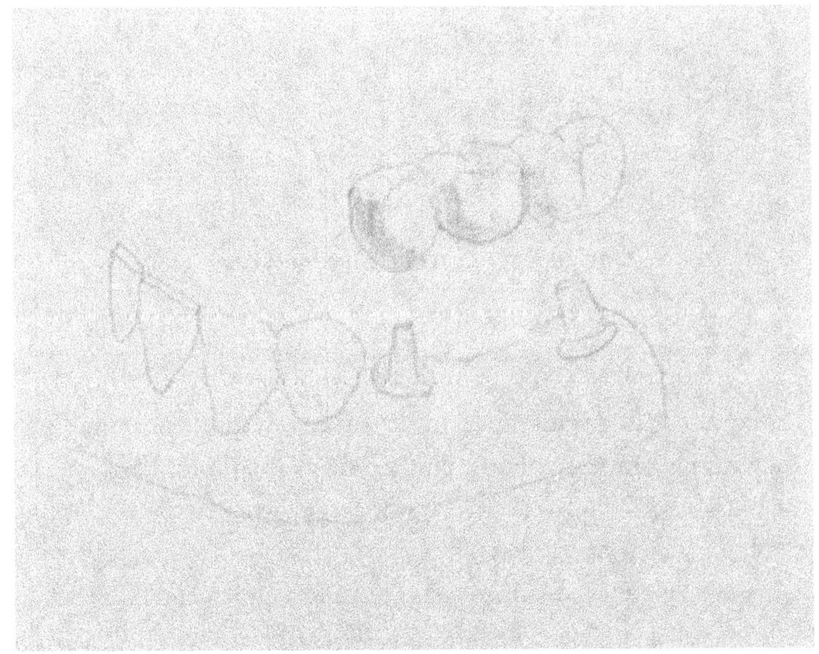

Fixed (cemented) bridge on natural teeth to replace one tooth: The natural teeth must be cut down to receive the bridge

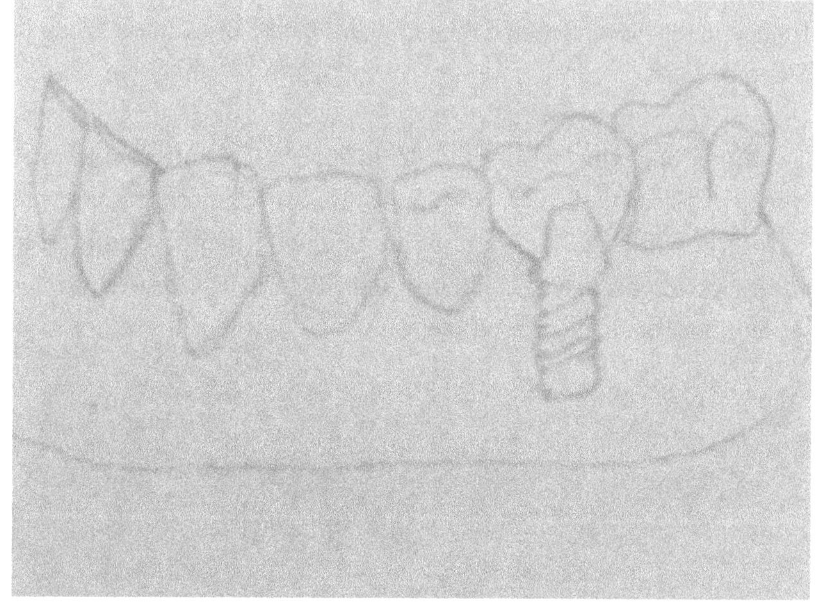

One implant to replace the molar tooth

They are still used sometimes to support removable dentures. When titanium implants are placed into a patient's jawbone, the fact that they fuse to the bone (**osseointegration**) is beneficial in preserving that bone which is attached. Otherwise, when teeth are removed, the natural healing process involves gradual loss of jawbone (known as resorption) over time, which eventually will interfere with function and possibly result in a situation in which insufficient bone remains in which to place implants. The gradual loss of jawbone also is a problem if dentures are constructed. The bone will gradually shrink and the dentures then become loose and ill-fitting. This can be particularly troublesome for the lower arch. Since the area on which the denture rests is somewhat "horseshoe-shaped", there is not much retention to begin with; this poor retention progresses as the bone loss increases over time.

Dental implants have become a common means of replacing missing natural teeth in patients of all ages. They are sometimes used in younger people (who have completed all jaw growth) due to traumatic loss of a tooth or multiple teeth. They can be used in all ages if the conditions are favorable, which I will expand on in upcoming chapters. The success rate is over 95%, depending upon which study is quoted, in healthy patients without certain medical conditions or habits. The success rate is slightly higher in the lower jaw, possibly related to higher bone density in the lower jaw. The lowest success is in the upper second (back) molar position (assuming most patients do not have their wisdom teeth, which are known as the third molars).

Alternatives to implant placement would be dentures (if all the teeth in a jaw are missing, or a partial removable denture if only some of the teeth are missing. The problems with removable appliances are multi-fold. Removable appliances are not as stable as fixed appliances or implants, because they partially rest on soft tissue which is movable. As the bone under the removable appliance shrinks over time, the appliance becomes more loose and doesn't fit as well. The removable partial denture has clasps and rests on natural teeth to help support it. As things change, undesirable forces can be placed on the natural teeth to which the partial denture is attached. In addition, bacterial plaque accumulates around the partial denture and adheres to the teeth. Over time, this can compromise the natural teeth. If a natural tooth around a partial denture requires future extraction (removal), depending upon the location in the arch and the design of the partial denture framework, the partial denture may require remaking if a key supporting tooth for the partial denture is one that is lost. In addition, if the partial denture design is incorrect, with respect to the location and types of rests and clasps, the natural teeth can become compromised and may eventually require extraction.

Implants are not generally joined to natural teeth, such as if two teeth side-by-side are missing. In other words, it is not recommended to bridge an implant to a natural tooth, because they are different entities. The natural tooth has slight movement due to the periodontal ligament surrounding it. The implant is essentially nonmobile, because it is fused to the bone. If they are joined, eventually the implant would be compromised due to the movement of the natural tooth it is connected to and resultant undesirable forces thereby transmitted to the implant.

The following alphabetically listed **definitions** will help patients to understand what I am talking about in the following text.

Abutment teeth: The natural teeth which support a fixed (cemented) bridge (anchor teeth)

Anterior: Toward the front of the mouth

Arch: This refers to a full upper jaw or lower jaw; the upper jaw is called the maxilla and is composed of less dense bone than the lower jaw which is called the mandible.

Bicuspids: (These are sometimes called premolars) are the teeth just forward of the molars. There are two per quadrant, or four per arch.

Bridge: A fixed (nonremovable) way to replace multiple missing teeth, or even a single missing tooth. With natural teeth, the bridge is cemented to the prepared (whittled down natural teeth). A bridge may also be placed on dental implants. With dental implants, bridges are held in place with precision screws specific to the manufacturer, or cemented.

Bruxism: Heavy grinding or clenching of teeth, usually during sleep; the patient is frequently unaware of this nighttime habit.

Buildup: A restorative process in which a hard composite material is used to replace the coronal (crown) part of the tooth that was destroyed by tooth decay

Canines: These teeth are adjacent to and forward of the bicuspids. These are sometimes referred to as "the cornerstones of the mouth" and are part of the **anterior** (front) teeth. There is one per quadrant, or two per arch.

Dental appliance: Refers to a removable object worn in the mouth that is made by a dental laboratory. It is usually for a teeth replacement option such as a denture, or partial denture, in which some natural teeth are retained to help support the artificial removable teeth. It may be temporary, such as a flipper.

Extraction: Removal of a natural tooth or implant.

Flipper: A temporary removable tooth replacement device that is used to mimic a tooth which is worn between the tooth removal and the final implant crown. This is made by a laboratory and is plastic (acrylic); it is usually reserved for front tooth/teeth or visible missing tooth/teeth areas.

Implant abutment: This is the intervening part between the implant body and the artificial tooth part or crown. This is placed with a miniature torque wrench specific to the manufactured brand of implant. This creates a tight, typically permanent connection between the implant body and the abutment. These are made of various materials: titanium, gold, ceramic materials such as zirconium.

Implant body: The "root" portion; Implants can be level with the bone, but sometimes have a polished portion (collar) which is slightly (1-2 mm) above the level of the bone.

Implant crown: The artificial tooth part that mimics a natural tooth in terms of function and appearance.

Incisors: These are the front teeth, sometimes called **anterior** teeth. There are two per quadrant, or four per arch

Keratinized tissue: A thicker, more resilient type of gum tissue surrounding natural teeth and on bone without teeth. This is desired around dental implants.

Molars: These are the large back teeth, used for crunching and grinding foods, and they are the largest teeth. There are two per quadrant, or four per arch. Most adults have a total of 28 -32 teeth in health. The wisdom teeth (or third molars) are normally absent; they are often extracted due to lack of jaw space. This leaves a full dentition of 28 teeth.

The neck of the tooth is also referred to as the cej, or cementoenamel junction. This is at or slightly above the jawbone level.

Occlusion: The way a patient's teeth fit together top to bottom. This requires precise attention to detail when restoring either natural teeth or implants. This is sometimes referred to as "the bite". If this is off or nonideal, it can result in damage to the restoration, fracture of either the restoration or root in a natural tooth. Poor occlusion may also result in fracture or loosening of the restoration on dental implant(s). If there is poor occlusion with implants, the natural opposing teeth (teeth in the opposite jaw that contact the implant restoration) may be damaged. The implant itself may lose its connection to the bone and become loose if the occlusion is too heavy. If the implant becomes loose, it is considered a failed implant and must be removed. Poor occlusion may also result in jaw joint problems, known as TMJ (temporomandibular joint) problems. You can feel this joint by placing your finger tips ahead of the ears when you open and close.

Osseointegration: Fusion of an implant to the bone

Partial denture framework: A specially designed cast metal framework to which artificial teeth and gums are attached.

Pontic: The false tooth in between the anchor teeth on a bridge, which replaces the missing tooth.

Posterior: Toward the back of the mouth

Prosthesis: some type of artificial teeth that are made by a laboratory at the dentist's prescription such as dentures, partial dentures (replacing only some teeth in an arch), or crowns/bridges on natural teeth or implants.

Quadrant: Each arch has two quadrants, right and left; this is one quarter of the jawbone for a patient

Resorption: Loss of jaw bone over time due to lack of teeth and pressure from a denture.

Restoration: The artificial parts that are used to either fix natural teeth with fillings or caps (cast gold or porcelain/ceramic material crowns) after removing decay, or the artificial parts placed on implants to return them to function and appearance as close as possible to nature.

Restore: To replace the missing natural parts of teeth or to place the parts on an implant that mimic as much as possible, the natural tooth/teeth.

Root canal: This is a procedure commonly done by a specialist called an endodontist, which involves removing the nerve and blood vessels inside the tooth, cleaning and shaping the internal part of the root (canal), and then filling the inside with special material that seals the tooth, allowing the natural tooth to be retained.

Suprastructure: A metal framework which is connected to the artificial teeth and gums in a hybrid prosthesis

Tooth anatomy or form: A natural tooth is composed of the root, which is situated in the jawbone of the patient. The crown of a natural tooth is the portion of the tooth one sees when looking in the mouth. This is covered with enamel and is the functional (chewing) portion of the tooth.

Zirconium: A very strong ceramic material that is white or tooth-colored and is preferred usually in anterior (front) tooth positions for the most ideal esthetic (appearance) result.

3

Implant Choices

When implants were first introduced in the United States, one of the first companies to supply them was a company named after Dr. Brånemark. This later morphed into what is now known as Nobel Biocare. Other large implant companies which have been considered leaders in implant research and development are Straumann (based in Switzerland), Astratech, Zimmer, and BioHorizons. The research and careful manufacturing techniques are important to the end result. The parts for tooth replacement: the implant, abutment, and crown must fit very precisely to increase the chance of longevity. Many patients have implants that have been in place successfully for 40-50 years. Millions of implants have been placed to date. It is not known exactly how many implants have been placed in the United States or worldwide, but they are thought to be used more in patients with a higher economic status. Dental insurance generally offers a benefit toward dental implant procedures, but it usually contributes far below the actual investment required. Dental "insurance" is really a misnomer. It would be better described as a dental "benefit", with a certain dollar contribution toward dental fees. In most cases and for all procedures, this has been the case for decades.

There are up to 75 or more implant companies, so things can be confusing. Many of these other implant manufacturers copy implants that were designed by the larger, research-based firms. These "copycat" companies claim that their parts are interchangeable with the original top five or six companies. It has been demonstrated that the "copycat" parts are not interchangeable in terms of precise fit and should not be used. They are sold and marketed to dentists at sometimes one third the cost of the top companies. My personal choice of top quality implants is Straumann, due to their strong clinical research, good reputation, and simplicity of design. Straumann is the #1 choice in the world. When new implant lines are developed by Straumann, the same instruments can usually be used to restore them. This is a big advantage in my opinion, and less confusing to the dentists who will be restoring (putting teeth on) them. A patient considering implants should inquire as to what type (manufacturer) the surgeon uses and why. There is usually literature which can be given to the patient about that particular implant.

4

Which Dentists Place Implants?

Patients may find that implants are now offered and placed by periodontists, oral surgeons, and general dentists. Traditionally, they were primarily placed by periodontists and oral surgeons, who have additional in-depth training in their specialty programs. Specialty training programs can range from three to five years following the completion of a 3-4 year dental school program. Most dental schools in the United States have a 4-year program (usually after 2-4 years of college) and confer either a DDS or DMD degree. There are a few dental schools which have a 3-year program leading to a DDS or DMD degree.

Periodontists are a natural choice for dental implant placement because they are skilled in soft tissue management and delicate, technical surgery; this is an important factor in dental implant surgery and the potential for longevity.

Oral surgeons trained in soft tissue management may also be an appropriate choice for implant surgery. Oral surgeons are trained in maxillofacial surgery which involves fracturing and repositioning the jaw(s), treating trauma such as jaw fractures, and removal of wisdom teeth, which is likely the most common procedure they perform.

General dentists who have taken extensive training in implant place-ment may be qualified also. Very fine general dentists may enroll in a course of several months duration in which they are treating live patients under supervision. These general dentists may wish to place implants.

Sadly, there are "weekend courses" or very limited-time investment courses for general dentists that do not necessarily qualify them as a favorable choice for the implant surgery. . Many of these courses are promoted by implant manufacturers which are interested in selling large numbers of implants to the dentists. The "copycat" type implants that are approximately one third the cost of the implants purchased from the large well-known companies in my opinion not a good choice. These are heavily marketed to general dentists.

General dentists place restorations on dental implants in the majority of cases. Prosthodontists are a group of specialist dentists that are very skilled in restoring natural teeth and dental implants. Quality is of paramount importance in implant dentistry. I look at implants as "replacing a missing body part" which will hopefully be in place for the lifetime of the patient. It doesn't make sense to cut corners with cheaper parts that have not undergone the vigorous research the top 5-10 companies do.

5

What are the Implant-Supported Options for Teeth Replacement?

Implants may be used for replacement of a single missing tooth, or for multiple teeth. Examples of a single tooth replacement would be if a patient has deep decay which has destroyed a large portion of the tooth, and resulted in a poor prognosis. The tooth might be able to be retained if a root canal is done, followed by a post and core buildup to restore part of the coronal part of the tooth and then a cap (crown). In this scenario, the decay may be very close to the bone, which would require a crown lengthening surgical procedure (normally performed by a periodontist) to allow the tooth to receive the restoration. Perhaps a better way to describe "crown lengthening is to refer to it as "gum shortening", which involves removing a small amount of bone around the tooth, then lowering the gum to this level. This exposes more of the coronal (top) part of the tooth, making it accessible to the dentist to restore and allow sufficient sound tooth structure for the gum to reattach. Each of these procedures is associated with a fee. When these fees are added together, they sometimes match or exceed the fees for a dental implant, abutment, and crown, the latter being much more predictable in terms of longevity.

The fact that the shape of the implant is different from the natural tooth shape presents some limitations. Most of these limitations can be overcome, with very careful restoration by the restorative dentist, usually a general dentist or a prosthodontist (specialist in crowns and bridges), either attached to natural teeth or implants. These may be removable. Since the dimension of the implant is usually smaller than the dimension of the natural tooth root, the shape of the crown (tooth) part attached to the implant must be carefully shaped at the level of the bone. It starts as a somewhat straight "emergence profile" at the level of the bone, then gradually expands to a normal sized tooth at the contact points between teeth and at the level of the chewing surface (see drawing below on the right). For this reason, it is important that the dentist restoring implants (putting the teeth on) is familiar with these concepts and uses a good laboratory to construct the teeth. I have seen many situations in which the laboratory constructed the crown with a very broad dimension at the level of the gum tissue. In the technician's mind, he/she is probably thinking the crown needs to look like a natural tooth, and by creating this shape, erroneously believes it will block food collection. If we were to look at an x-ray of a crown like this, it looks like "a lollipop on a stick". The abrupt horizontal angles off the implant actually create a food trap and patients do not appreciate having to dislodge food after every meal (drawing on the left). It is somewhat counter-intuitive to start with a small dimension at the level of the implant, but it is necessary. Not every dentist understands this.

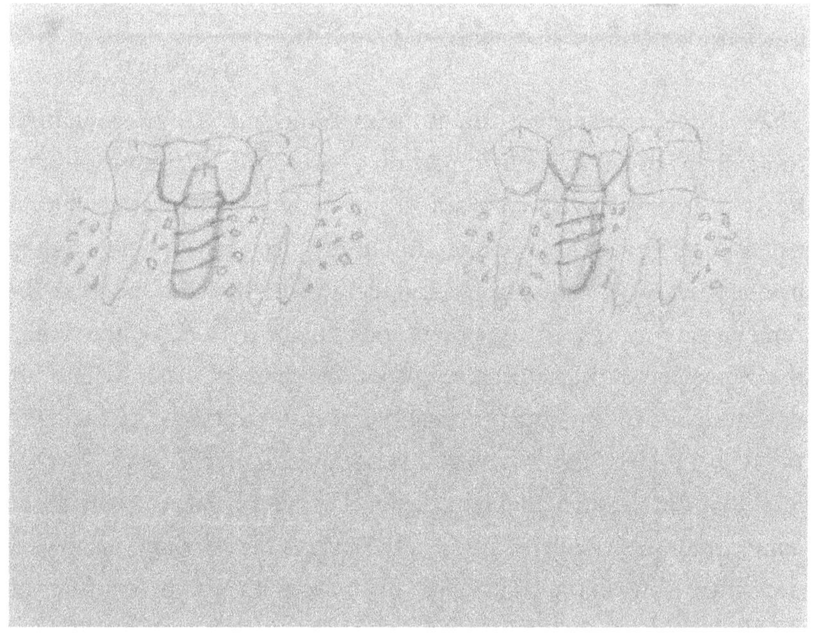

Improper shape of crown on implant Correct shape of crown on implant

Individual implant crowns or bridges may be used for implant restorations. These are normally held in place with tiny screws specific to the type of implant, with a special torque wrench also specific to the implant brand used. It is important that the restorative dentist understands thoroughly the requirements for the specific implant which was placed. If a screw-retained implant crown becomes loose from the abutment, it must be reattached with a <u>new</u> implant screw specific to the manufacturer of that implant. Cement is sometimes used to retain implant bridges, especially in the front part of the mouth, due to the angle of the jaw. There are certain risks with restorations (single crown or bridge) cemented to implants, so cementation is preferably used only when the angle of the jaw necessitates this. This is most common in the front (anterior) part of the mouth. The potential problem with cemented crowns or bridges on implants has to do with excess cement that may be left. This can be particularly harmful if a certain type of cement known as a glass ionomer is used. This cement sets very hard under the gum margin; excess cement is difficult if not impossible to remove once it sets. It does not appear on x-rays, so it may not be obvious to the dentist that excess cement was left. The implant restorative parts have a precision fit, so there is very little room for the cement. If excess cement is left below the gum, it eventually contributes to bacterial accumulation and bone loss around the implant, which may cause failure of the implant over time. This may not become obvious until 3-4 years have passed following implant placement. For these reasons, I usually recommend using temporary cement, which is easier to remove excess of, and which allows the ability to remove the crown if necessary. There are techniques that the dentist can use to minimize excess permanent cement. These techniques were published by two prosthodontists (Wahdwani and Pineyro) from Bellevue, WA. several years ago.

There are now options for offset screws with some implant systems that still allow screws even if the jaw bone is angled. This is the most common implant restoration in the U.S., replacing one or two teeth at a time.

Other types of implant restorations involve a **combination of implants and removable appliances**, most commonly full dentures. Full dentures are artificial teeth which replace all the teeth of either the top arch or lower arch, and sometimes both. When dentures can be attached to dental implant abutments (which are attached to dental implants anchored in the bone), they are much more stable and function much better than full dentures alone. Generally 2-4 implants are placed in the jawbone. After a healing period of 2-4 months, special abutments may be placed which correspond to special attachments placed in the denture, making it much more stable and less movable. This is most commonly beneficial for the lower jaw, because the shape of the denture is somewhat "horseshoe shaped" to fit over the lower jaw and avoid the floor of the mouth and tongue. The lower jaw undergoes resorption or bone dissolution after the teeth are removed. This is a progressive process. If a patient needs to lose all of her/his teeth in the lower jaw, it is best to consider two implants early on. The more resorption or loss of bone that occurs over time, the less chance there is of having sufficient bone in which to place implants.

Implants are generally not used to help support maxillary (upper) dentures, because the upper denture covers the roof of the mouth, and therefore is fairly retentive in most instances. Some patients however, do not want the acrylic of the denture to cover the roof of the mouth, so 4 to 6 implants may be placed in the upper jaw, and the palatal acrylic of the denture may be removed, so it appears more like a horseshoe, which is supported solely by the implants. When significantly large amounts of bone are missing in the upper jaw due to resorption, this option can be a very good one, and the patient has the ability to remove the denture to clean the implants daily with their toothbrush and other aids.

The other thing that happens after loss of all of the teeth in a jaw, particularly the mandibular (lower) jaw is a change in the nature of the tissue covering the jawbone. It can become thin and mobile, particularly when a denture rests on it for years. Once implants are anchored in the jawbone, they help retain the bone and resist additional resorption. When placing implants, it is most desirable to have what is known as keratinized tissue surrounding an implant neck at the level of the bone.

It is more resilient in terms of bacterial accumulation, is easier to clean around and is believed to be important in long-term retention of dental implants. Sometimes it is necessary for the surgeon to correct the lack of sufficient keratinized tissue before or after implant placement by means of a plastic surgical gingival (gum) graft.

Hybrid Prostheses are also known as fixed detachable implant restorations; they can be removed by the dentist once/year to check the integrity of the implants and screws, but they are not removed by the patient (fixed). These can be a very nice option for patients, because they are screwed onto a bar or suprastructure that is attached to the implants. Many patients prefer this type of restoration because they do not remove the teeth from their mouths; they are taught to clean around the prosthesis. This may feel more natural to them, and they never go without the facial support that the appliance provides. A colleague and prosthodontist who was a leader in these types of restorations was Dr. Earl Ness. He was guiding and restoring these types of treatment over 35 years ago, long before it became popular 15-20 years ago.

Hybrid prostheses are a type of restoration that require a team of trained individuals to master: the dentist planning the case with the surgeon, and a laboratory technician skilled in these techniques. These are the types of restorations that are used when companies advertise to patients that they can receive new teeth the same day the teeth are removed. There are some important features that must be understood with this type of restoration.

All the teeth in the particular arch (top or bottom) must be removed in order to create this type of restoration. So this type of treatment is reserved for those with advanced bone loss around most teeth, or very poor esthetics related to crowding, decay, stain.

The teeth which are put on the implants at the time of placement are only temporary, and must be replaced in approximately 6 months. Sometimes the temporary teeth may not be attached to the implants at the same time as implant placement, because the bone is too weak (this is tested with a torque device at the time of implant surgery).

Usually with this type of treatment, large amounts of jawbone are removed in order to create the minimum distance of 15-17 mm between the bone and opposing teeth locations. This space is necessary for the parts required in this hybrid prosthesis.

It is best to complete one arch at a time. After complete healing, the second arch can be done.

The cost of this type of restoration is approximately $35,000-$50,000 per arch, which includes the surgery, dentist's restoration, and laboratory fees.

Careful design and a team approach are imperative for this type of treatment.

6

Approximate Cost of Implants and the Restorations

There is quite a variation in fees for these specialized procedures. Fees tend to be higher in larger cities. For a single tooth replacement (one implant, one abutment, one crown), the fee may be approximately $5000-$6000. If a bridge were used to replace the single tooth, it would be a 3-unit bridge, because it is anchored on either end with a single natural tooth and the missing tooth is soldered in the middle. This replacement for the missing tooth is called a pontic. This requires cementation to the natural teeth. Performing oral hygiene is more difficult because the dental floss must be threaded under the pontic to adequately clean the teeth supporting the bridge. The cost of this restoration is similar to the cost of the implant/crown option. It is a more immediate solution and can be completed in 3-4 weeks. The dental insurance industry however, estimates that the average lifetime of a fixed bridge (attached to natural teeth) is 7 years. Decay can develop at the margins of the bridge, or fractures can occur. When a fixed bridge requires replacement, slightly more tooth structure is removed on the teeth on which the bridge is cemented; the existing bridge must first be removed. This sometimes involves cutting the bridge off. If a root canal treated tooth is one of the anchor teeth, it can develop a root fracture. This is a less conservative means of replacing teeth in most cases, because it involves cutting down or removing natural tooth structure, the purpose being to anchor the bridge which has the soldered missing tooth.

As mentioned previously, The cost of the fixed detachable (or Hybrid) type of restoration is approximately $35,000-$50,000 per arch, which includes the surgery, dentist's restoration, and laboratory fees.

If removable appliances are anchored by 4-6 implants per arch, the cost is markedly less than the hybrid prosthesis (perhaps half to ⅔ less), because planning time is reduced, and fewer parts are required. In addition, there is less laboratory time needed.

7

Planning for Implants

If an implant is planned, the site for the implant must first be developed or healed. When a tooth is extracted, it takes approximately 4 months for the extraction site to heal before an implant is placed. There is another healing period following placement of 2-4 months, and then the crown can be fabricated by the laboratory after the dentist provides the necessary records: impression of the implant and record of the bite (occlusion). Sometimes a temporary tooth may be attached to the implant at the time of implant placement.

Sometimes a bone graft is required at the time of extraction due to very thin bone. In my opinion, it is generally best to have the surgeon who will be placing the implant perform the extraction, so that the need for a bone graft may be assessed. It is best to place the bone graft at the time of extraction. Sometimes a moderate amount of bone can be lost at the time of extraction. This can be due to infection which causes bone loss, either from extensive decay or a fractured tooth root. At times the root is fused to the bone; if the bone is very thin, part of the socket may be lost. In this case, special membranes to temporarily contain the bone graft and platelet rich plasma or other biologic materials may be used to establish good bone for an implant. Platelet rich plasma is offered in some periodontist and oral surgeon offices. It involves drawing a small quantity of the patient's own blood, and placing it in a special centrifuge. The centrifuge spins the blood-containing tubes at a specific rpm in a matter of minutes, which separates the layers of blood. The platelet-rich layer is separated out with micropipettes and is used at the surgical site. This layer is helpful because the platelets (which aid in blood coagulation) also contain several growth factors which aid in healing and minimization of discomfort.

There are some difficult situations which can be present in planning a site for an implant. Teeth which require extraction in order to develop the site for an implant can be challenging. For instance, the upper first bicuspid tooth is one of the more difficult teeth to remove without trauma. It has two very thin roots which can easily break if extreme care is not taken. The bone is typically very thin around these roots, and it is important to preserve the bone.

Sometimes the teeth requiring extraction are very close to an adjacent tooth in which case the bone between those two teeth is very thin. It is important to get the tooth out without harming the adjacent tooth. In addition, the tooth requiring extraction may be root canal treated, which makes the tooth more brittle; there is a greater chance the tooth is fused to the bone. In many cases, a combination of these factors is present. For these reasons, each situation must be managed with specific techniques for the optimal outcome.

8

Standard of Care for Optimal Outcome

Proper diagnostic information is imperative when planning for dental implants. Diagnostic impressions are initially obtained and made into diagnostic casts (study models) which can be mounted on a device which mimics the opening and closing of the mouth. These are mounted as closely as possible to the patient's occlusion (bite) and requires obtaining a bite registration (a record obtained at the dental chair which allows proper mounting of the models). Depending upon how many implants are required, the diagnostic records can be more involved, such as in the case of a hybrid prosthesis. Team planning between the dentist restoring the implant and the periodontist/surgeon is important prior to extraction of any teeth. The periodontist may direct the restorative dentist to provide a "stent" to guide the desired location of the implant. This is a clear plastic removable device, usually made by a dental lab. In compromised or crowded situations, this is important to the end result. The following is an example. In this case, since there was extreme crowding, I requested that the dentist have his lab prepare a "diagnostic wax-up", which is what one would like the result to be, and determine the ideal location for the dental implant(s). Even though two teeth were missing, the plan was to place one implant, then have the lab construct a "cantilever" pontic. This is the missing lateral incisor tooth, which is attached to the main implant crown on the central incisor. A flipper was used as an interim appliance. The lab-fabricated stent was used to guide the location of the implant.

Tooth #8 hopeless; crowding

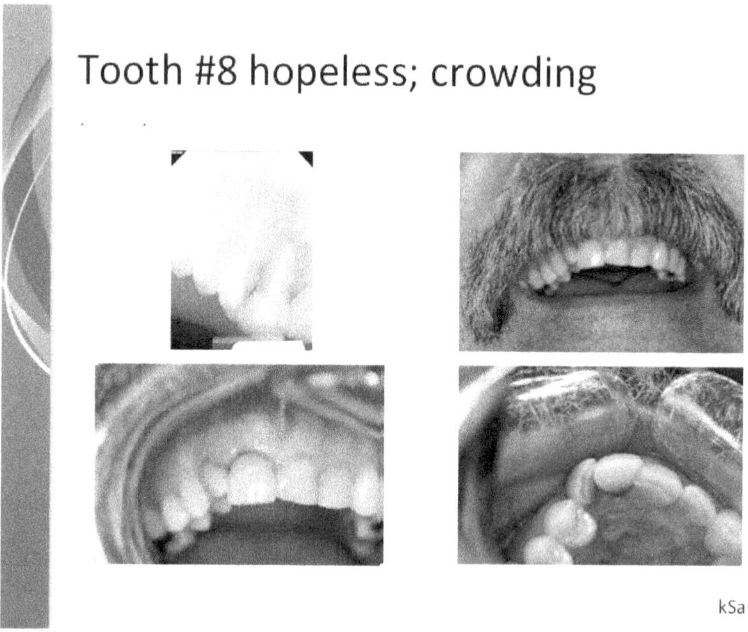

Surgical Implant Stent and "Flipper"

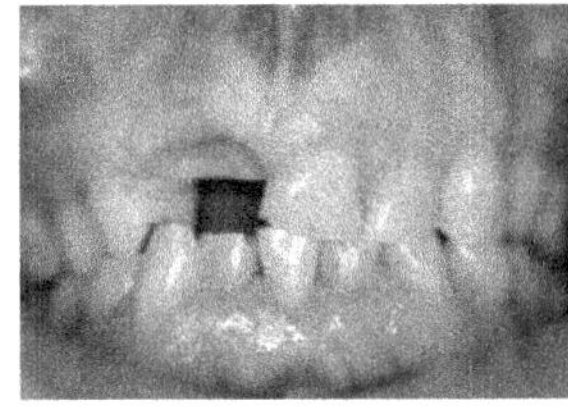
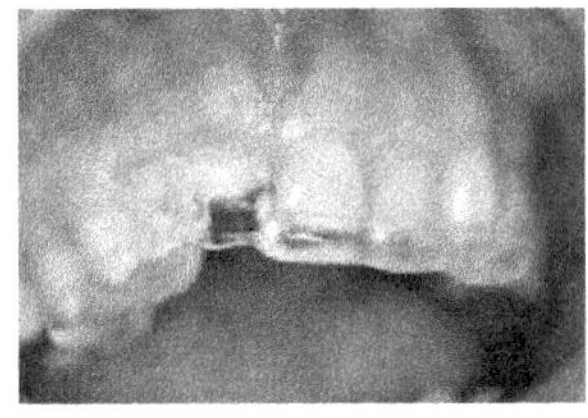
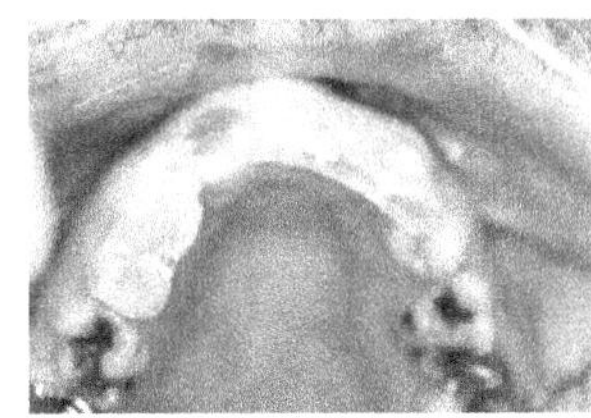
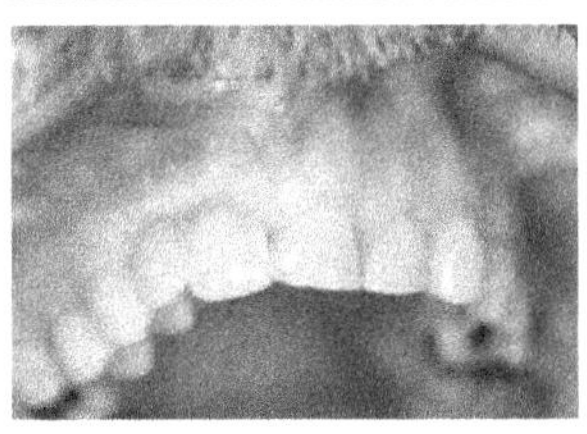

kSa

Straumann Bone Level Roxolid TiZr Implant placement with stent

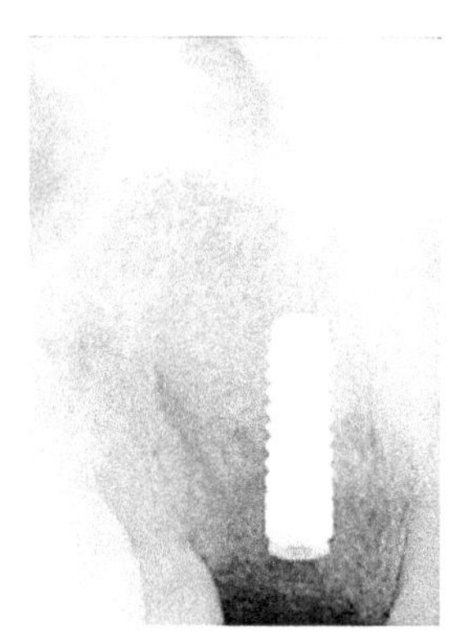

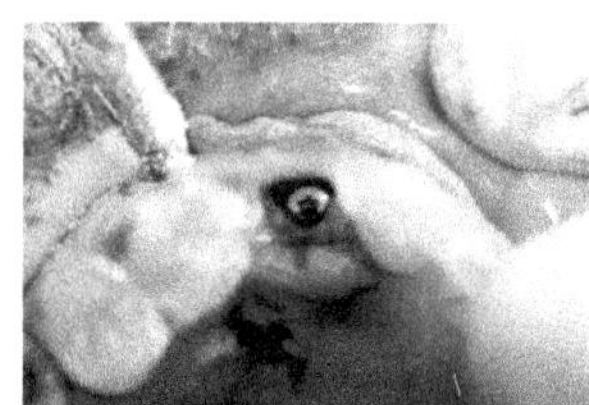

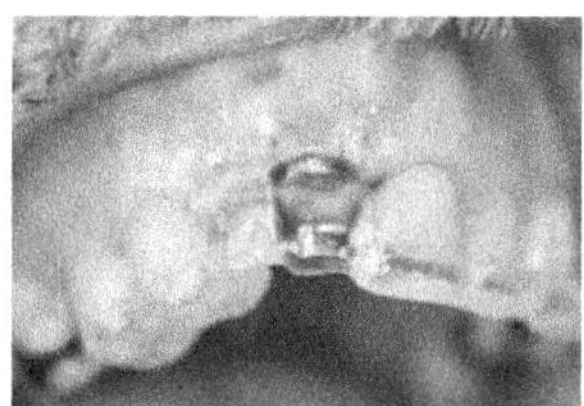

kSa

Final

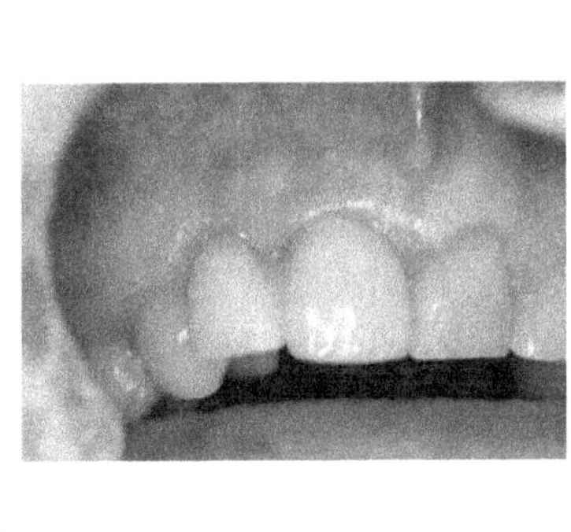
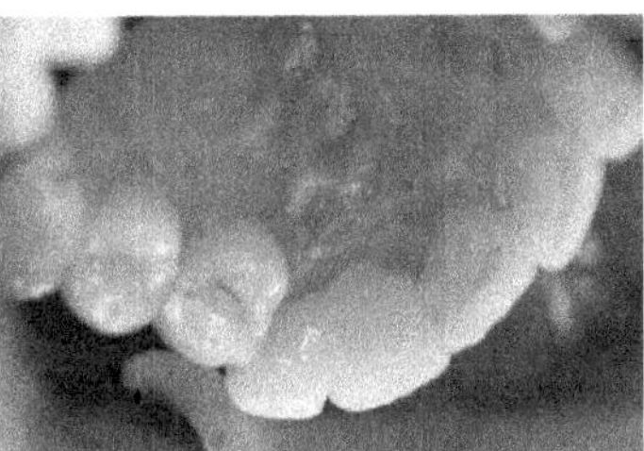

Intraoral dental x-rays are obtained, and in most cases a 3-dimensional CT scan which is specific to the jaws and dental needs. The CT scan allows the surgeon to view the jawbone in 3 dimensions in order to evaluate the width of the bone, angle, and anatomical structures. Certain anatomical structures which must be avoided in the placement of dental implants include nerves (such as in the lower portion of the lower jaw) and sinuses (air spaces) in the upper jaw. Sometimes, unexpected findings are revealed, such as fractured off root tips, foreign bodies, or cysts. These special CT images allow the surgeon to evaluate whether the patient is a candidate for implant(s) and if additional procedures such as bone augmentation will be necessary. Not all patients are good candidates for dental implants due to quantity and quality of bone or other reasons. This must be discussed before any treatment is rendered. When there is advanced vertical bone loss, it is acceptable to have the lab use pink porcelain in the final restoration to mimic the gum tissue.

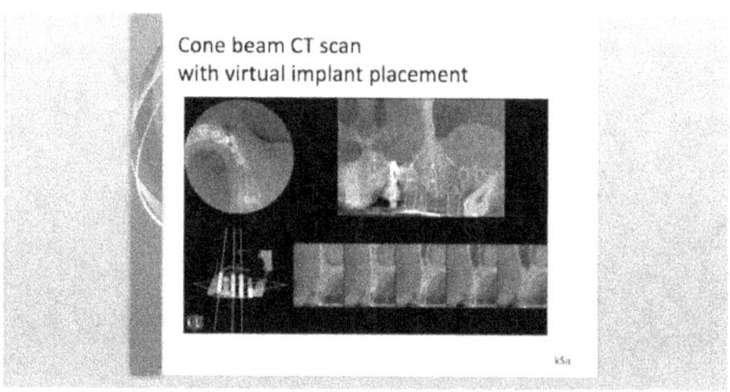

In the upper jaw, sinuses (air spaces) are part of the normal anatomy. When upper teeth are removed and not immediately planned for replacement, the sinus can drop down, which ultimately allows for less vertical height of bone. In this case, it should be determined prior to surgery that a sinus lift may be necessary. A CT scan is of utmost importance in the planning process. There are several ways in which a sinus lift can be accomplished. The most straightforward method is to gently vertically lift the sinus and place bone graft material underneath the raised sinus membrane. Sometimes this can be done at the same time as implant placement, but if there is a severe lack of vertical height of bone, it is a two-stage procedure, in which the sinus lift/bone graft is done first, then another CT is obtained following 6-8 months of healing.

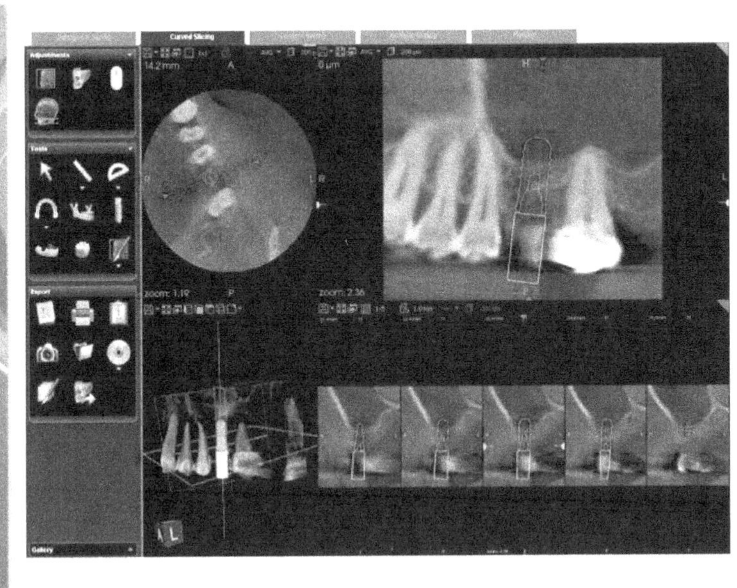

In this CT scan example, the upper right portion of the image demonstrates insufficient vertical height of bone for an implant. Using the imaging software, a dental implant of the ideal size and brand is placed in the site. This is denoted by the green outline of an implant. In this case, the implant would project up into the sinus (air space), so a sinus lift would be required. This is illustrated on the following x-rays.

Crestal Sinus Lift with simultaneous implant placement

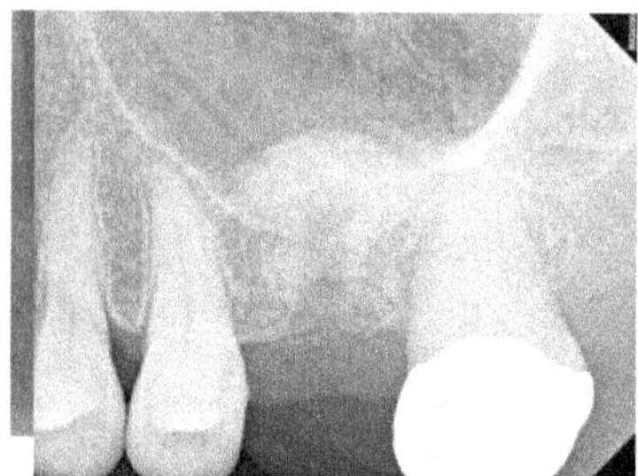 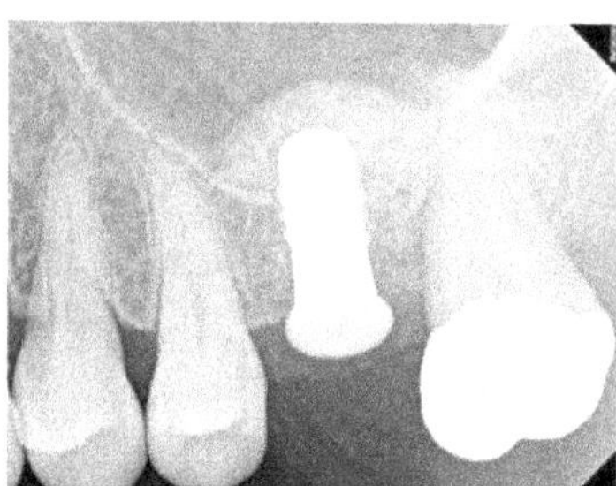

If the diagnostic records indicate that a patient is a good candidate for placement of dental implant(s), it is critical that careful placement be planned, with sterile implant surgery instruments and implant motor, and that the dental assistant is knowledgeable about his/her role during the surgery. Personally I believe that a sterile set-up is optimal (sterile drapes on all counters in the room, sterile instruments, and sterile irrigating solution). Sterile hair covers, surgical masks, and protective eyewear should be worn by all in the room. I also recommend a sterile scrub-in prior to donning sterile gowns and sterile gloves. Nothing should touch the implant as it is being readied to be delivered into the prepared site in the bone. Only the patient's bone should contact the implant, which is delivered with precise rpm speed and irrigation (sterile water coolant). In most cases, a "healing abutment" (a temporary screw placed on the implant which is slightly above the gum level is placed to protect the top of the implant during the healing phase of 2-4 months. Sometimes a temporary acrylic crown is placed, but it may not be in contact with the opposing teeth and cannot be used for chewing. Closure of the site is carefully done with special sutures that don't encourage bacterial accumulation. One common choice of suture is a "GORE-TEX type" or eptfe (polytetrafluoroethelene). Polyglactin (Vicryl) sutures are another choice. These are strong sutures with antibacterial properties. Although they are absorbed (dissolved by the body) in 56-70 days, they are typically removed by the surgeon in 7-14 days. Silk sutures should <u>not</u> be used, because they are braided and can draw bacteria into the tissue. Non-steroidal antiinflammatory drugs such as ibuprofen or prescription diflunisal can be given right before starting the surgery, provided the patient is a candidate for this drug type. This prevents pain afterwards. Careful preoperative and postoperative written instructions, as well as verbal instructions are given to the patient and an additional family member (this is mandatory if the patient has received any type of sedation). There is rarely a need for postoperative pain medication. The patient needs to avoid chewing near the implant site. If the implant is in an upper front tooth position, there is usually a temporary removable prosthesis (sometimes called a "flipper") which the patient can use during healing that mimics a tooth. Alternatively, a temporary crown is placed in an esthetic area that shows.

Sometimes additional bone must be created at the time of implant placement for a successful implant healing in which the entire "root portion" of the implant is surrounded by bone. In this case, bone material and sometimes additional biologic materials are put around the implant to fill a void, and generally intentionally covered up by the gum tissue for optimal healing. After the healing period (typically 4 months), the implant is surgically uncovered and the healing abutment is placed. The implant is now ready for restoration.

Some surgeons will use an ISQ device (Implant Stability Quotient) to assess the stability of an implant and determine the best time to restore it. This patented device works by Radio Frequency Analysis to predict implant stability.

9

What are Some of the Risk Factors with Implant Success?

Smoking is not recommended. Although smoking is not an absolute reason to avoid implants, it is a risk that the implant may not fuse to the bone, and would therefore be considered a failure. I prefer to treat non-smokers with implants, or minimally have the patient discontinue smoking 3 weeks prior to surgery and 6 weeks after. Some patients may need help with this smoking reduction, and may use nicotine patches or other temporary aids.

Diabetes, either type I or type II is a risk factor in implant surgery. The A1C (glycated hemoglobin) is the ideal medical test which is checked in diabetic patients. Controlled diabetics (blood sugar is under good control and monitored by the patient's physician) can do well with implants, but this diabetic control must be maintained. It is important to reduce interference with diabetics' food consumption routine during the surgical phase, particularly if the patient is taking medications to lower the blood glucose.

Another risk factor for implants is a habit of heavy teeth clenching, known as bruxism. For these patients, when the final crown is placed on the implant, it is important that it is very slightly out of occlusion (no contact), and that it be checked regularly because the opposing teeth may drift into contact again. I would recommend an upper hard acrylic custom night guard (fabricated by a dental laboratory on the direction of the dentist). Although most patients would not be aware of nighttime grinding or clenching, it is extremely common and can lead to implant failure. I suggest an upper night guard for most implant patients as a preventive measure. The dentist should give the lab detailed instructions for the fabrication of the night guard. It should ideally be a heat-processed hard acrylic, tooth-borne appliance, with even centric contacts on anteriors and posteriors, and have canine guidance. In communication with the dentists, I include these detailed written instructions which can be transferred to the dental lab. Patients need to be instructed to bring their night guard to any dental appointment in which the bite (occlusion) may be adjusted, or if a filling or crown is done, because the night guard will likely require adjustment to maintain proper fit.

Certain medications may pose a risk factor for long term implant success. It is important to inform your dentists of all medications that are taken, as well as a history of medications. Patients who have a history of taking bisphosphonates such as Fosamax or Alendronate are at risk of improper bone healing and a serious bone infection, medication-induced osteonecrosis. This is a serious infection which does not respond well to treatment. Large amounts of jaw bone may be lost with the infection. These bisphosphonate drugs are commonly used for post-menopausal osteoporosis. However sometimes this category of medications is used to treat breast cancer. In this instance, the drug is administered intravenously and not all of the drug is eliminated over time. These patients in my opinion are not good candidates for dental implants.

There is some recent research suggesting that oral bisphosphonate drugs do not necessarily result in more implant failure. I still suggest caution and do not recommend surgical treatment while the patient is actively taking the drug. There are alternative drugs used to treat bone density problems that patients could discuss with their physicians. One suggestion is the drug class monoclonal antibodies. One common example of these is Prolia, an injection approximately at 6 month intervals. In between injections, there is a safer window in which implants may be placed at less risk than with bisphosphonates.

Drugs which have been shown to affect successful implant retention are proton pump inhibitors (such as omeprazole). These are very common drugs which are prescribed to millions of Americans; they reduce stomach acid Many of these drugs can be obtained without a prescription. There is a higher implant failure rate in patients taking these medications.

There is also a potential problem with certain antidepressants known as SSRIs (serotonin reuptake inhibitors). The mechanism is unknown, but there is a higher implant failure rate in patients taking these drugs.

Interestingly, some blood pressure medications actually result in enhanced bone remodeling and osseointegration. This blood pressure reducer is a RAS (renin angiotensin system) inhibitor.

Another risk to implant success would be poor or improper oral hygiene on the part of the patient. Using implements that poke, such as toothpicks around an implant can cause failure. Overaggressive, improper flossing can also cause implant failure.

10

The Importance of Maintenance

I t is very important that patients perform proper daily oral hygiene with careful flossing and brushing as demonstrated by their hygienists or dentists. They should also be seen every three months for maintenance (teeth cleaning) by their hygienists or dentists. The implants need to be assessed at these maintenance appointments for cleanliness, lack of gum tissue inflammation, and lack of mobility. The occlusion should also be checked. If any mobility is detected, there may be a loose crown, or the implant may be loose. An x-ray is normally taken to help with the assessment. Sometimes, with a screw-retained crown, it is simply a loose screw. In this case, the screw and crown would be removed, and a new screw would be placed with the miniature torque wrench. The abutment may be loose, which would be reattached with a new screw if it is screw-retained. The implant manufacturer (at least the large most popular companies) have technical support divisions which can help diagnose a problem and suggest solutions. The fact that minor problems like this can occasionally occur is another reason for dentists to select a popular name brand implant company. Sometimes patients have come into the office with an implant problem, but the implant is not recognizable. This adds complexity to solving the problem if the implant manufacturer cannot be easily determined. There are resources available to help discover the type of the implant, but it may be difficult to find parts. Using a well-known manufacturer is very helpful in avoiding problems of this type, adding to a satisfying and predictable result.

11

Conclusion

Implants have revolutionized dentistry in terms of restoring patients to natural function and appearance. This is important for patients' overall health and confidence. Gone can be the days of poor nourishment due to the inability of a patient to chew food appropriately. There is no upper age limit for implants for patients with good health and adequate bone. Dental implant placement requires attention to detail, gathering adequate preoperative clinical records and team planning. It is very rewarding and a wise investment. It has been my honor to help patients achieve their goals of teeth replacement to restore function and esthetics.

I hope you have found the information presented in this book to be useful in terms of education about the dental implant process and what your choices are for replacement of missing teeth.

I would very much appreciate it if you kindly post a review on Amazon.

12

Notes: Questions for your dentist

13

Notes: Questions for your Periodontist or Surgeon

14

Notes: Medications you are taking that may influence the outcome for dental implants

15

Notes: Questions you may have for your dental insurance (benefits) company

<h1 style="text-align:center">16</h1>

<h1 style="text-align:center">References</h1>

Branemark. (1969). Intra-osseous anchorage of dental prostheses: I. Experimental studies. *J Plastic Reconstr*.

Buser. (2017). Modern implant dentistry based on osseointegration: 50 years of progress, current trends and open questions. *Periodontol 2000*.

Christiansen. (2012). Why are dental implants not used more in the United States? *JADA*.

Cullum, Deporter. (2015). Minimally Invasive Comprehensive Treatment: Case Studies. In *Minimally Invasive Comprehensive Treatment: Case Studies* (p. Chapter 21). Wiley.

Jofre. (2013). Influence of minimally invasive implant-retained overdenture on patients' quality of life: a randomized clinical trial. *Clin Oral Res*, 1173–1177.

Saravi. (2021a). Impact of renin-angiotensin system inhibitors and beta-blockers on dental implant stability. *Int J Implant Dent.*

Stavropoulos. (2018). The effect of antiresorptive drugs on implant therapy: Systematic review and meta-analysis. *Clin Oral Implant J.*

Tarnow (Ed.). (2014). J. Perio. In *Journal of Periodontology* (85th ed., Vol. 11, pp.1475–1477).Wiley.

Wahdwani. (2009). Technique for controlling the cement for an implant crown. *J Prosth Dent.*

Wang. (2021). The peri-implant phenotype and implant esthetic complications. Contemporary overview. *Journal of Esthetic.*

Afterword

Many of the situations we encounter in clinical practice demand careful preoperative planning and consultation with all dentists involved, before treatment commences. It can be very traumatic for a patient to lose a natural tooth or multiple natural teeth. Dedicated professionals are available to assist in restoring ideal function and appearance. This is a team approach, and patients should always feel free to ask questions and obtain explanations that they understand.

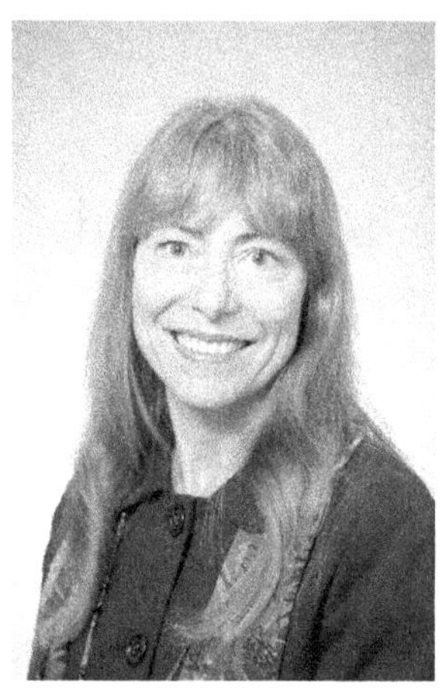

About the Author

Dr. Kathleen Stambaugh is a periodontist in the State of Washington. She grew up in the Bay Area, northern California and attended U.C.Berkeley and UCLA before obtaining her DDS (Doctor of Dental Surgery) degree from UCLA. She then completed a general practice residency at the V. A. Medical Center in San Diego. She returned to Los Angeles and earned a specialty certificate in Periodontics from the Greater Los Angeles V.A. Medical Center. She is a Board Diplomate in Periodontics and is actively serving in various roles with the American Academy of Periodontology (AAP). Dr. Stambaugh practiced in West Los Angeles with her husband Dr. Roger Stambaugh, until the Northridge earthquake in 1994 destroyed their medical building. She started a new practice in Washington at that time and has been honored to educate and treat her periodontal patients. The information in this book is her own opinion and is not sponsored by the AAP.